you're a fighter not a quitter!

M. y. cux

THE
BREAST
CANCER
GPS

A Guided Journal to Navigate
Your Way Through
Breast Cancer

THE BREAST CANCER

GPS

ISBN: 978-1-7367038-0-9

DEDICATION

Thank you to Jamie Aronson Tyus for helping me when I was first diagnosed and providing me my starting point for this journal. For all my Pink Sisters who have been there and given me advice and tips to fight the fight and to my family and friends for supporting me with their love.

Dear Pink Sister,

I am sorry you must join us in this club but know that you are not alone. There are others before you who have fought and conquered. We have all been in your shoes and know it is scary. Where to start? What to ask? Do I remove my breasts? What do I do next? I have provided a starting point for you: A list of questions to ask breast surgeons, plastic surgeons, oncologists and radiologists. Please add to these questions so that it will help you understand and help you with your decisions. Be kind to yourself as you navigate through your treatments. You are an inspiration to all. You are a fighter, a warrior and most of all a SURVIVOR!

This Journal belongs to:

_____

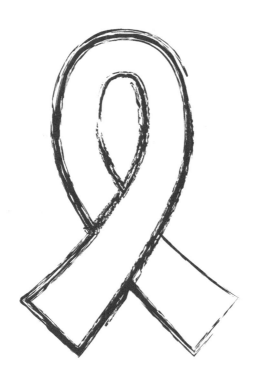

Questions, Questions, Questions...

Who can remember it all?

Every doctor has a sheet for you to fill out. What is your medical history? Any family members have cancer and list who they are and the relationship to you. Who is your emergency contact? What medications are you on? Blah Blah Blah...the list goes on. Who can remember all of this? Within these pages you will be able to write everything down. Bring this journal with you to appointments so you have it handy to relay the information.

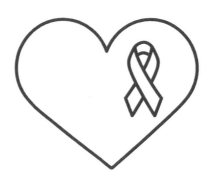

Name: _____

DOB: _____

Blood type: _____

Height: _____

Weight: _____

Emergency Contact:

_____

_____

_____

_____

_____

Allergies and/or Reactions:

_____

_____

_____

_____

_____

Surgeries and dates:

_____

_____

_____

_____

_____

Complications if any:

_____

_____

_____

_____

_____

Family Medical History:

Mother's Side:

RELATIVE	ILLNESS

Family Medical History:

Father's Side:

RELATIVE	ILLNESS

List of Prescribed Medications:

Drug Name	Strength	Dose	Prescribed by

List of Over-the-Counter Medications/Supplements:

Drug Name	Strength	Dose	Prescribed by

List of Tests Since Cancer Diagnosis

Scan/Test	Date	Location	Results

Doctors and Numbers:

Primary Care: _____

Number: _____

OB/GYN: _____

Number: _____

Dermatologist: _____

Number: _____

_____   _____

_____   _____

_____   _____

_____   _____

_____   _____

_____   _____

what
do
YOU
choose to be
a victim of
Cancer?
or a survivor of
Cancer?

Now let us get to the doctor questions, shall we?

We know you need to pick your team and you want to get the right one. Breast surgeon...who will do what you want? Are they listening to you? Plastic surgeon - are you getting implants or doing a DIEP flap? What are your options? Your oncologist will be with you for at least 10 years so make sure you like them! *DO NOT* be afraid to change doctors if you are not happy...this is your life...you are in control. I would recommend taking someone with you to help you interpret as you will probably only hear half of it because all you can think about is "I have this tumor in me and I want it out NOW!" Take notes...or even record if the doctor will let you so you can go back and listen.

Abbreviations...
what does it all mean?

AC - Chemo drug: Doxorubicin (Adriamycin) aka Red Devil, and Cyclophosphamide (Cytoxan).

CMF - Cyclophosphamide/Methotrexate/Flourouracil

FEC - Flourouracil/Epirubicin/Cyclophosphamide (chemo cocktail)

TtC - Taxotere/Carboplatin

BC- Breast Cancer

BX- Biopsy

SNB - Sentinel Node Biopsy

DX - Diagnosis

IBC - Inflamatory Breast Cancer

IDC - Invasive Ductal Carcinoma

ILC - Invasive Lobular Carcinoma

DCIS - Ductal Carcinoma in Situ

IDCIS - Invasive Ductal Carcinoma in Situ

LCIS - Lobular Carcinoma in Situ

ANC - Ancillary Node Clearance

ALND - Axillary Lymph Node Dissection

ER- Estrogen Receptor

PR- Progesterone Receptor

LN - Lymph Node

Lx - Lumpectomy
MX - Mastectomy
UMX- Unilateral Mastectomy
BMX - Bilateral Mastectomy
DMX - Double Mastectomy
DIEP - Deep Inferior Epigastric Perforator
MPBC - Metaplastic Breast Cancer (not to be confused with metastatic breast cancer) - an aggressive rare form of breast cancer.
IMBC-Invasive Micropapillary Breast Carcinoma--
METS - Metastatic
SE - Side Effect
ANC - Absolute Neutrophil Count
WBC - White Blood Count
RBC - Red Blood Count
LE - Lymphedema
PICC line - Peripherally Inserted Central Line
PORT - Port-a-cath
Mammo - Mammogram
U/S - Ultrasound
ECHO - EchocardiogramRADS - Radiation/RadiotherapypCR- pathological complete response
NED - no evidence of disease
NEAD - No Evidence of Active Disease. Used for stage 4.
Onc - Oncologist
PS - Plastic Surgeon

BS - Breast Surgeon
NP - Nurse Practioner
GP- General Practioner
PCP - Primary Care Physician
GS - General Surgeon
BRCA = BRCA1 and BRCA2
(Breast Cancer genes 1 and 2)
BARD1 another BC gene

Breast Surgeon Questions:

The surgeon should explain to you the difference between a lumpectomy and a mastectomy. Either the surgeon or your oncologist will want you to get gene testing done... are you BRCA positive? This could determine between a lumpectomy vs a mastectomy if not a double mastectomy.

- What is a lumpectomy vs mastectomy?

- Will there be drain tubes and what are those?

- How long are those in for?

- Where would you make the incision?

- If doing reconstruction what needs to be done? Expanders?

- Do you leave skin?

- Does the plastic surgeon also do anything during this first surgery?

- If not doing reconstruction and I want to stay flat... will you honor that? I do not want skin left, dog ears... I want it to be clean and flat. I do not want to have to go back and do more surgery because you left extra skin.

- If having a mastectomy (or double) do you have a physical therapist you recommend to help after surgery? (this will help with range of motion)

- If I am BRCA positive what does that mean?

- Should I also have a hysterectomy?

- Does the surgery come first or chemotherapy if it is needed?

What other questions do you have?

_____

_____

_____

_____

_____

_____

_____

_____

_____

_____

_____

_____

_____

_____

_____

_____

_____

_____

_____

_____

Notes from Breast Surgeon

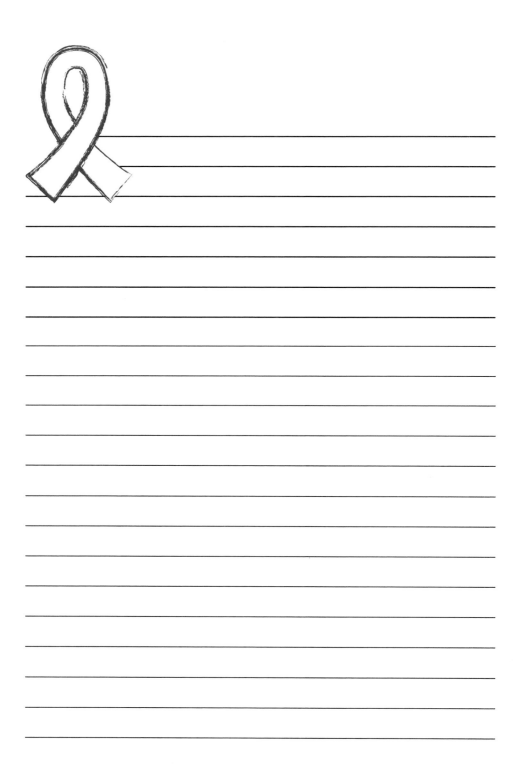

Plastic Surgeon Questions:

If you plan on getting reconstruction which way do you want to go? Do you want implants? Do you want to do a DIEP flap?

- Will the reconstruction happen at the same time of the mastectomy?

- How do implants work?

- How many surgeries will I need?

- Do the implants need to be changed out after so many years?

- What is DIEP flap?

- Am I a candidate for it?

- What does it all entail?

- Expanders?

- Are those necessary? What do they do?

- Do the expanders go under the muscle or can it go over?

- How many surgeries with a DIEP flap?

- How long am I under for implants vs DIEP flap?

- Will I need blood transfusions?

- How long in the hospital?

- Drain tubes? Will those be needed and what exactly is that?

- How long are they in for?

- How long is the recovery?

- What is needed at home?

- Side effects?

- When can it be done?

- Do you recommend waiting for a period of time?

- If I must do chemo or radiation will the surgery interfere?

- Will more surgery need to be done because they shrank or with radiation the skin is too tight?

- I understand there are different phases. Phase 1 is the reconstruction. Phase 2: to fix areas...give examples

- What are the pros and cons?

- With DIEP flap what if the skin fails and does not take? Then what happens?

- Nipple reconstruction?

- What kind of changes over time should I expect?

- Will I need future surgery to lift for example?

- What happens if I gain or lose weight?

- When would I be able to do normal activities? Drive, lift kids, etc?

- What type of clothing can I wear?

- Instead of doing the reconstruction and I remain flat... would liposuction help with the thighs and buttocks to make my frame more proportionate?

- What does that all entail?

- Recovery? What is needed?

- Can the fat come back?

- What do I need to do to maintain?

- Do you have referrals of women I can speak with?

What other questions do you have?

_____

_____

_____

_____

_____

_____

_____

_____

_____

_____

_____

_____

_____

_____

_____

_____

_____

_____

_____

Notes from Plastic Surgeon

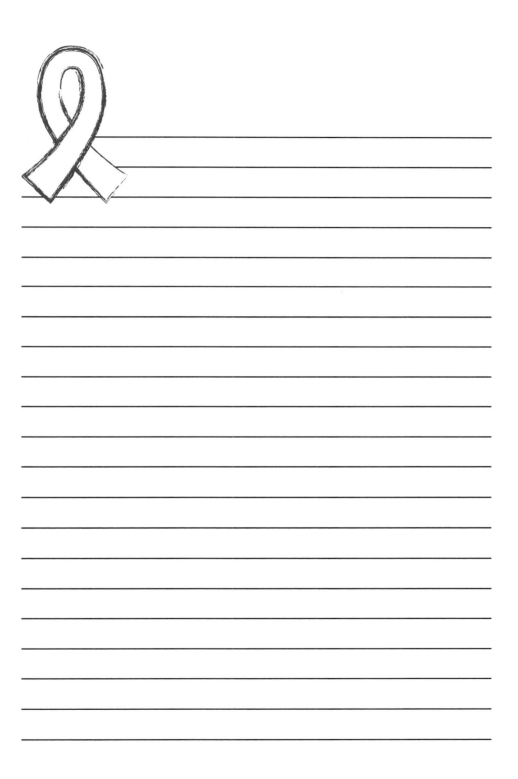

Oncologist Questions:

Know some of these questions cannot be answered until you have your surgery, but let the doctor explain everything. This doctor will be with you for a long time. In the beginning, during treatment, you will see them weekly. When completed with treatment, every 3 months and so forth until you are done long term.

- Is the estrogen- receptor positive or negative?

- Is the progesterone- receptor positive or negative?

- HER2 positive or negative?

- What is the stage?

- What is the size?

- What is the oncotype DX?

- CT scan/PET scan – check whole body for cancer?

- How often do you do scans?

- How quickly is it growing?

- What grade is my tumor?

- What is my lymph node status?

- How likely to recur?

- If I take both breasts, do I still need to do chemo or radiation or both?

- If a lumpectomy, what is the process with that? Still radiation/chemo?

- If I must do chemo would I be able to use cold caps?

- What do you feel is the best course of treatment for me?

- Should I be changing my diet? exercise?

What other questions do you have?

_____

_____

_____

_____

_____

_____

_____

_____

_____

_____

_____

_____

_____

_____

_____

_____

_____

Notes from Oncologist

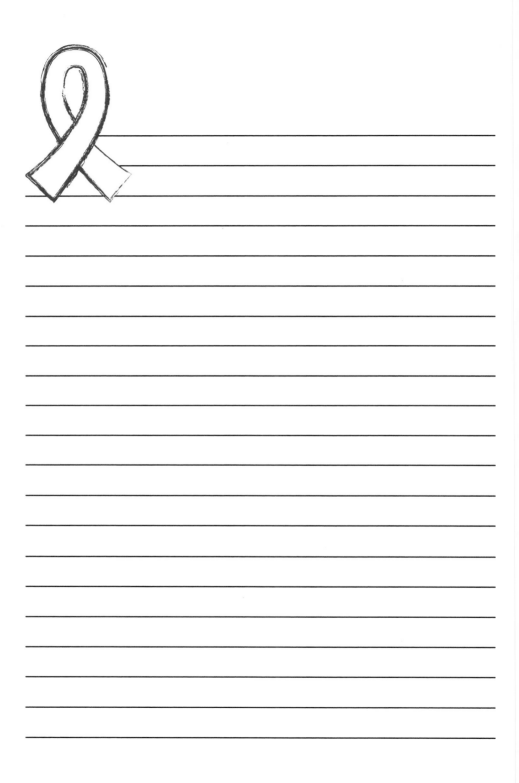

Radiologist Questions:

Depending on what you decide, lumpectomy vs mastectomy your treatment can vary. For example, there is brachytherapy which is aggressive and is shorter (1 or 2 sessions a day for maybe 5 days) than your everyday radiation which can last 3-5 weeks. This doctor will inform you the best treatment plan for your type of cancer.

- What is brachytherapy?

- What are the benefits of this type?

- How often do I come for this?

- Is this only for lumpectomies?

- For the regular type of radiation - how often is this?

- What are the side effects to both?

- What can I put on my skin to prevent burning?

- How often should this be done?

- Am I able to swim?

- Am I able to lift?

- Am I able to exercise?

What other questions do you have?

_____

_____

_____

_____

_____

_____

_____

_____

_____

_____

_____

_____

_____

_____

Notes from Radiologist

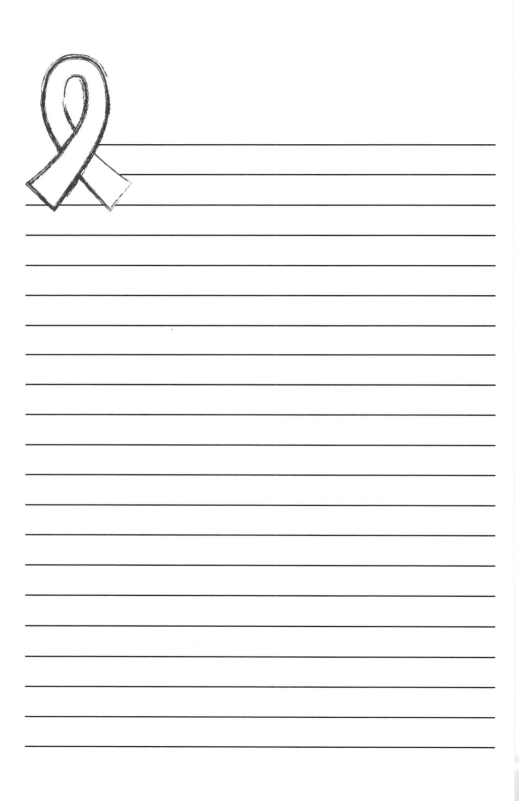

Tips and Tricks from other Pink Sisters

We have been in your shoes and along the way others have helped one another get through this and you will get through this too! Do you have your financials in order? Wills? Financial and Medical Power of Attorney, Living Will, beneficiaries, etc. In the meantime, some helpful tips and tricks to get you through the hurdles.

Surgery:

In hospital: (if you spend the night)
- Arnica 30C two weeks before surgery and two weeks after to help with bruising (Sprouts, Whole Foods)
- Phone charger
- iPad or other tablet
- Books
- Robe
- Lip balm
- Button up shirts (you will have drains so you won't be able to lift your arms)
- Stretchy pants
- Slip on shoes

At home recovery:

You need to be taken care of and not the other way around. Accept offers of service, such as cleaning, cooking, babysitting, errands, rides to follow-up doctor appts, help with changing of dressings on sutures, help with emptying and recording of drains.

Mastectomy:

- Recliner - you will probably be sleeping in it for a few weeks to a month.
- Carpenter's apron to hold drains
- Lanyard to hold drains
- Robe with inside pockets to hold drains
    (find what is right for you)
- Ginger ale and ginger pills for nausea
- Neosporin or Bacitracin for suture and drain holes
- Comfy non-slip socks
- Slippers
- Shower chair - depends on your doctor but you may not be allowed to fully shower just yet.
- Bathing wipes
- Mastectomy pillows
- Maternity pillow - once in bed this was great to use to not let you roll over
- Small pillows all over when you are in the chair
- Blankets
- Back Scratcher

- Soft pajamas that button in the front or zip up as you will not be able to lift your arms for a few weeks.
- Heated neck pad
- A basket or tray to keep at bedside (or by the recliner) to keep necessities close at hand.
- Lots of time to catch up on movies, shows, and books! Enjoy the quiet time!

Lumpectomy:
This is an easier recovery, but you can still use everything above. You still need to take care of yourself.

Chemotherapy:

- Hydrate, Hydrate, Hydrate! Some even say when chemo is done have them hydrate you.
- Lidocaine - to put on your port 45 minutes prior so you don't feel the needle
- A blanket
- Books, magazines, coloring books
- iPad or other tablet
- Slippers or warm socks
- Some women have the Neulesta shot the next day and can be achy - Claritin or Aleve can help
- Anti-nausea medications
- Supplements - probiotics, Vitamin C, Vitamin D, hair, skin and nails.

ALWAYS CHECK WITH YOUR DOCTOR BEFORE TAKING SUPPLEMENTS, OVER-THE-COUNTER MEDICATIONS, OR OTHER MEDICATIONS TO SEE IF THEY WILL INTERFERE WITH TREATMENT. USE THAT ON-CALL DOCTOR NO MATTER WHAT.

- Try to eat what you can
- You may need protein shakes
- Check with nutritionist as chemo can affect your body in different ways so certain foods can help
- Stool softeners as constipation can occur
- Fiber to help with your gut
- Be concerned with a fever over 100.5, call your doctor or go to the ER.
- Prescription mouthwash if you get sores
- Biotene for dry mouth
- Make sure to floss and keep up with dental cleanings
- Essential oils can help with nausea, headaches, relaxation

YOU KNOW YOUR BODY. DO NOT BE AFRAID TO ASK YOUR DOCTOR FOR HELP!

Radiation:

- Hydrate, Hydrate, Hydrate!
- No lotions, perfumes, deodorant prior to your treatment
- Undershirts to wear afterwards so the lotion does not get all over your clothes
- 100% aloe gel (4x a day)
- Calendula lotion (put on after aloe gel)
- Prescription lotion (2x a day - right after treatment and at night)
- You may burn from it so make sure you lotion all the time to try to prevent It.
- Stretching to prevent tightness

How are you feeling?

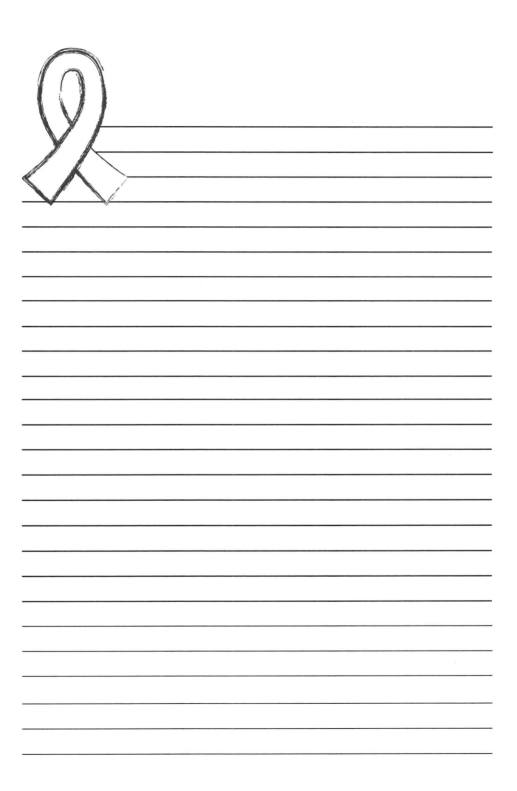

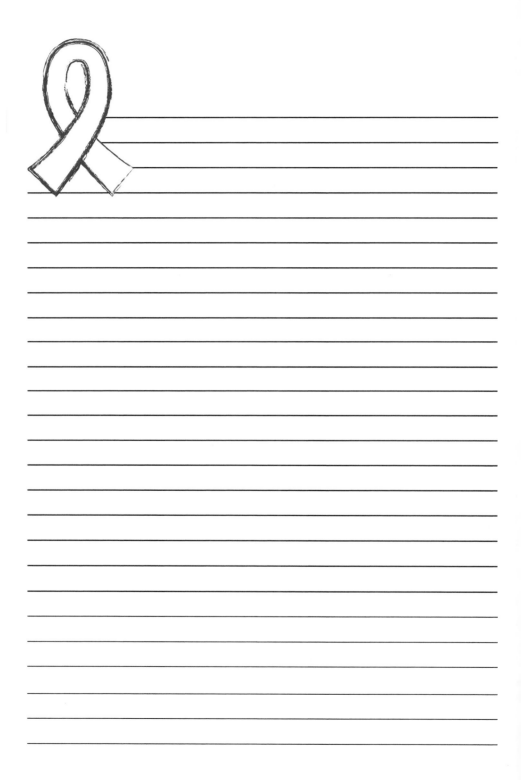

Resources

Medical bills, house bills, groceries, housecleaning.. they all add up. Even if you are working it still takes a toll on you. Check with your employer, can you go on FMLA? Ask the nurse or patient navigator or the social worker for grants in your state relating to breast cancer. You may need to apply a few times, do not get discouraged just keep applying. Pharmaceutical patient assistance programs are also available once treatment is done to help with ongoing medications or shots.

Make sure you have documentation on hand (like your medical history, bills and/or employment documentation). Grants usually need to be applied between the 1-5th of the month. Below are just a few, check your state for more.

American Cancer Society 800.227.2345
Cancercare.org
nationalbreastcancer.org
www.cancerhorizons.com/free-stuff
www.knittedknockers.org
https://cleaningforareason.org
breastcancer.org

More Resources

Support Groups

This is a very difficult time for you, your significant other and your family. It is okay to be emotional. It is okay to lash out. There are groups out there to help you throughout this time. There are support groups locally, online and one-on-one. I highly recommend reaching out and asking for help.

Support Groups in My Area

_____

_____

_____

_____

_____

_____

_____

_____

_____

_____

_____

_____

Cancer changes you, makes you slow down and re-think things. What are some things you have always wanted to do? Start your life list and do them!

MY LIFE LIST

THINGS I WILL DO THIS YEAR   *DONE*

_____   ☐

_____   ☐

_____   ☐

_____   ☐

_____   ☐

_____   ☐

_____   ☐

_____   ☐

_____   ☐

_____   ☐

Week of ____/____/____   **My daily activities
during chemo/radiation**

Monday

_____
_____
_____
_____

Tuesday

_____
_____
_____
_____

Wednesday

_____
_____
_____
_____

Thursday

_____
_____
_____
_____

Friday

_____
_____
_____
_____

Saturday

_____
_____
_____
_____

Sunday

_____
_____
_____
_____

Week of ___/___/___

Monday

_____
_____
_____
_____

Tuesday

_____
_____
_____
_____

Wednesday

_____
_____
_____
_____

Thursday

_____
_____
_____
_____

Friday

_____
_____
_____
_____

Saturday

_____
_____
_____
_____

Sunday

_____
_____
_____
_____

Week of ___/___/___

Monday

_____
_____
_____
_____

Tuesday

_____
_____
_____
_____

Wednesday

_____
_____
_____
_____

Thursday

_____
_____
_____
_____

Friday

_____
_____
_____
_____

Saturday

_____
_____
_____
_____

Sunday

_____
_____
_____
_____

Week of ___/___/___

Monday

_____
_____
_____
_____

Tuesday

_____
_____
_____
_____

Wednesday

_____
_____
_____
_____

Thursday

_____
_____
_____
_____

Friday

_____
_____
_____
_____

Saturday

_____
_____
_____
_____

Sunday

_____
_____
_____
_____

Week of ___/___/___

Monday

_____
_____
_____
_____

Tuesday

_____
_____
_____
_____

Wednesday

_____
_____
_____
_____

Thursday

_____
_____
_____
_____

Friday

_____
_____
_____
_____

Saturday

_____
_____
_____
_____

Sunday

_____
_____
_____
_____

Week of ___/___/___

Monday

_____
_____
_____
_____

Tuesday

_____
_____
_____

Wednesday

_____
_____
_____
_____

Thursday

_____
_____
_____

Friday

_____
_____
_____
_____

Saturday

_____
_____
_____
_____

Sunday

_____
_____
_____
_____

Week of ___/___/___

Monday

_____
_____
_____
_____

Tuesday

_____
_____
_____
_____

Wednesday

_____
_____
_____
_____

Thursday

_____
_____
_____
_____

Friday

_____
_____
_____
_____

Saturday

_____
_____
_____
_____

Sunday

_____
_____
_____
_____

Week of ___/___/___

Monday

_____
_____
_____
_____

Tuesday

_____
_____
_____
_____

Wednesday

_____
_____
_____
_____

Thursday

_____
_____
_____
_____

Friday

_____
_____
_____
_____

Saturday

_____
_____
_____
_____

Sunday

_____
_____
_____
_____

Week of ___/___/___

Monday
_____
_____
_____
_____

Tuesday
_____
_____
_____
_____

Wednesday
_____
_____
_____
_____

Thursday
_____
_____
_____
_____

Friday
_____
_____
_____
_____

Saturday
_____
_____
_____
_____

Sunday
_____
_____
_____
_____

Week of ___/___/___

Monday

_____
_____
_____
_____

Tuesday

_____
_____
_____
_____

Wednesday

_____
_____
_____
_____

Thursday

_____
_____
_____
_____

Friday

_____
_____
_____
_____

Saturday

_____
_____
_____
_____

Sunday

_____
_____
_____
_____

Week of ___/___/___

Monday

_____
_____
_____
_____

Tuesday

_____
_____
_____
_____

Wednesday

_____
_____
_____
_____

Thursday

_____
_____
_____
_____

Friday

_____
_____
_____
_____

Saturday

_____
_____
_____
_____

Sunday

_____
_____
_____
_____

Week of ___/___/___

Monday

_____
_____
_____
_____

Tuesday

_____
_____
_____
_____

Wednesday

_____
_____
_____
_____

Thursday

_____
_____
_____
_____

Friday

_____
_____
_____
_____

Saturday

_____
_____
_____
_____

Sunday

_____
_____
_____
_____

Week of ___/___/___

Monday

_____
_____
_____
_____

Tuesday

_____
_____
_____
_____

Wednesday

_____
_____
_____
_____

Thursday

_____
_____
_____
_____

Friday

_____
_____
_____
_____

Saturday

_____
_____
_____
_____

Sunday

_____
_____
_____
_____

Week of ___/___/___

Monday

_____

_____

_____

_____

Tuesday

_____

_____

_____

_____

Wednesday

_____

_____

_____

_____

Thursday

_____

_____

_____

_____

Friday

_____

_____

_____

_____

Saturday

_____

_____

_____

_____

Sunday

_____

_____

_____

_____

Week of ___/___/___

Monday

_____
_____
_____
_____

Tuesday

_____
_____
_____
_____

Wednesday

_____
_____
_____
_____

Thursday

_____
_____
_____
_____

Friday

_____
_____
_____
_____

Saturday

_____
_____
_____
_____

Sunday

_____
_____
_____
_____

Week of ___/___/___

Monday
_____
_____
_____
_____

Tuesday
_____
_____
_____
_____

Wednesday
_____
_____
_____
_____

Thursday
_____
_____
_____
_____

Friday
_____
_____
_____
_____

Saturday
_____
_____
_____
_____

Sunday
_____
_____
_____
_____

Week of ___/___/___

Monday

_____
_____
_____
_____

Tuesday

_____
_____
_____
_____

Wednesday

_____
_____
_____
_____

Thursday

_____
_____
_____
_____

Friday

_____
_____
_____
_____

Saturday

_____
_____
_____
_____

Sunday

_____
_____
_____
_____

Week of ___/___/___

Monday

_____
_____
_____
_____

Tuesday

_____
_____
_____
_____

Wednesday

_____
_____
_____
_____

Thursday

_____
_____
_____
_____

Friday

_____
_____
_____
_____

Saturday

_____
_____
_____
_____

Sunday

_____
_____
_____
_____

Week of ___/___/___

Monday
_____
_____
_____
_____

Tuesday
_____
_____
_____

Wednesday
_____
_____
_____
_____

Thursday
_____
_____
_____

Friday
_____
_____
_____
_____

Saturday
_____
_____
_____

Sunday
_____
_____
_____
_____

Week of ___/___/___

Monday

_____
_____
_____
_____

Tuesday

_____
_____
_____
_____

Wednesday

_____
_____
_____
_____

Thursday

_____
_____
_____
_____

Friday

_____
_____
_____
_____

Saturday

_____
_____
_____
_____

Sunday

_____
_____
_____
_____

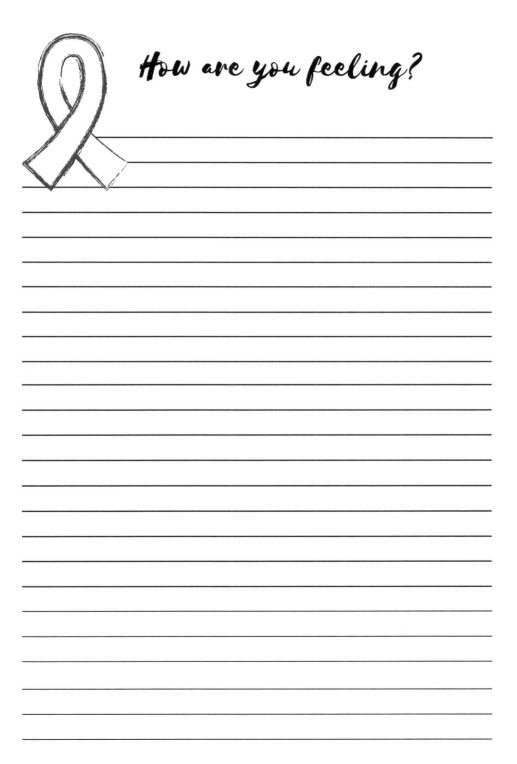

How are you feeling?

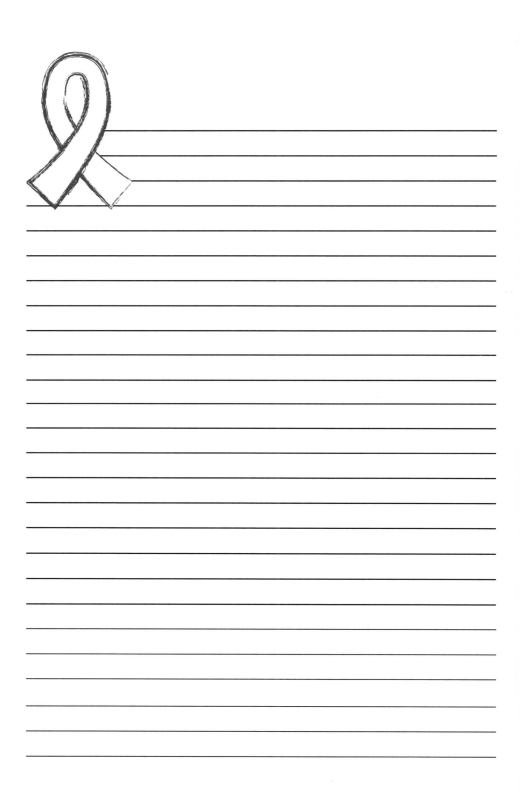

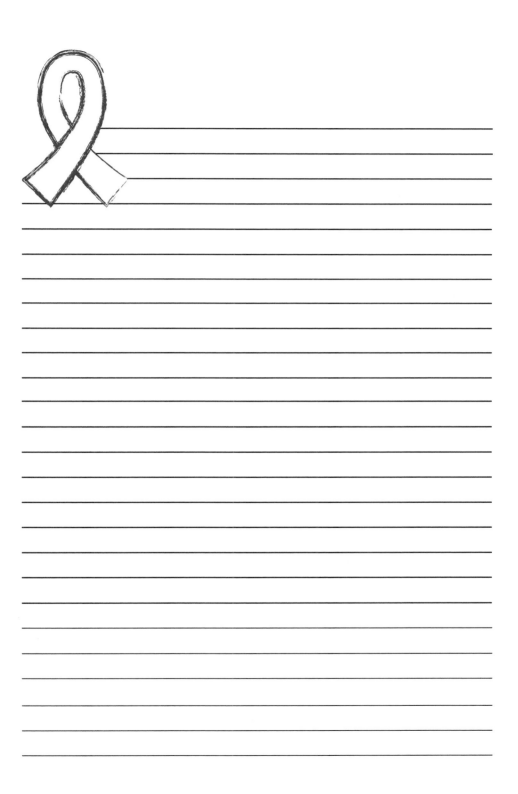

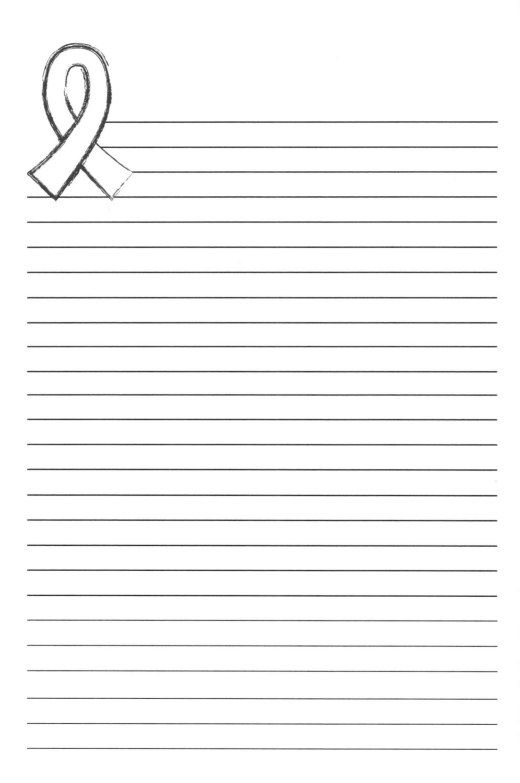

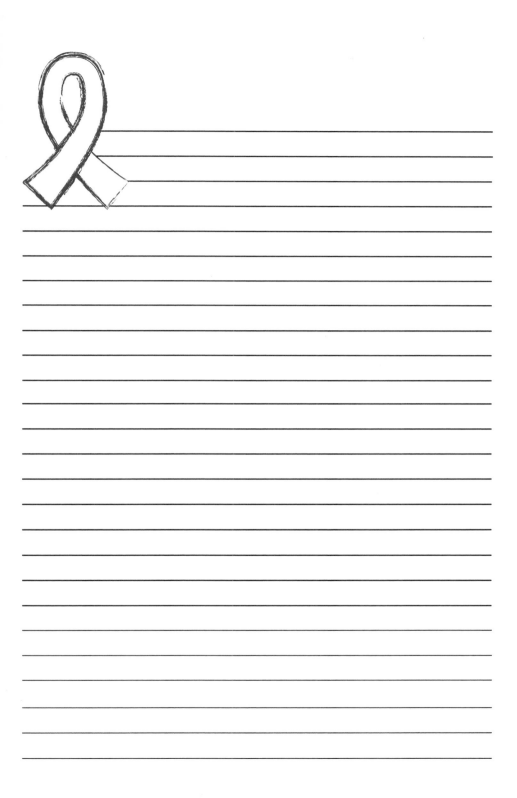